Valerian. Or, the Virtues of That Root in Nervous Disorders; and the Characters Which Distinguish the True From the False. By John Hill, ... The Second Edition

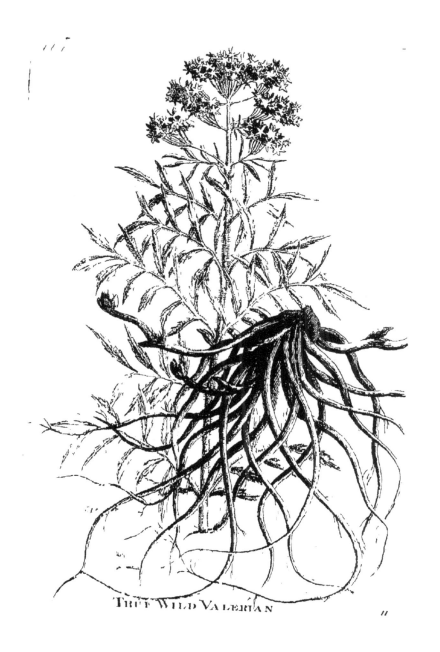

TRUE WILD VALERIAN

_II_

VALERIAN.

OR,

The Virtues of that Root

IN

NERVOUS DISORDERS;

AND

The CHARACTERS which diſtinguiſh the TRUE from the FALSE.

By JOHN HILL, M. D.

Illuſtrated with FIGURES.

THE SECOND EDITION.

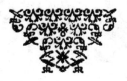

LONDON.
Printed for R. BALDWIN in Paternoſter-row.
M DCC LVIII.
[Price One Shilling.]

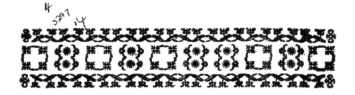

VALERIAN.

CHAP. I.

Of the Nature of the Root.

PHYSICANS find uncertainty in the effects of Valerian ; and the medicine has loſt ſome part of its credit : I beg they will hear the following reaſons. When the cauſes of that uncertainty are ſhewn, the remedy will be eaſy.

By the application to theſe purpoſes botany becomes uſeful to mankind : and 'tis a misfortune the ſcience is ſo little cultivated in England. Some ſhould enquire into the ſtate of drugs; and determine with equal freedom againſt ignoᵣance and fraud: but this cannot be expected from the phyſicians, for the ſuperior care of health does not allow them leiſure : the age is not deficient in HIPPOCRATES's; but there wants a *Cratevas*.

By VALERIAN, we underſtand the root of the large wild plant of that name : its ſuperior virtues having baniſhed the other kinds. This grows on heaths, by rivers, and in woods : but

B 2

does,

does, not in all these places, equally possess its virtues. When in perfection, it is highly aromatick : we know that quality depends in a great measure, on sun and air; and is impaired always, and often destroyed utterly, by shade and water. Therefore the roots of Valerian which grow upon dry hills and sun-burnt heaths, possess its virtues in the highest degree; and such only should be used in medicine. Unhappily the plant is more common by waters ; and the roots are in wet places larger, and more easily taken up A pound of these is brought into the shops for every dram of the other : and as they are greatly inferior in their qualities, the physician is disappointed who depends on them.

Not only the virtues, but the stature, colour, and whole aspect of the plant are altered by this watery nourishment: and though in reality the two kinds are only varieties, occasioned by the different soil, yet they are so considerable, that Ray and others have given the mountain Valerian, a distinct place in their catalogues ; accounting it a different species from that growing by waters.

In woods it assumes a form distinct from both; and propeily is of a middle kind between them. Its virtues are also of a middle character ; inferior to those of the heath, and superior to those of water Valerian.

The excellence of Heath Valerian is such, that no other should be used ; and there is enough of it for the demand. The distinction is obvious, as will appear by the succeeding
ing

ing characters : and as the term WILD belongs equally to the wood and water kinds, as well as to the true, it may be proper to diftinguifh that hereafter by the name HEATH VALERIAN.

C H A P. II.

Defcription of the Plant, and of the frefh Root.

THE root is compofed of many fibres joined to a fmall oblong head. The ftalk is erect, round, jointed, hollow, and toward the bottom, reddifh. The leaves ftand in pairs; and each is compofed alfo of many leffer leaves joined to a long rib, with an odd one at the end. The flowers are fmall and reddifh; and they ftand in large tufts at the tops of the ftalk and branches. Each flower is formed of one piece; and is tubular at the bafe, fwelled out on one fide, and cut into five parts at the rim. It has no cup: and it is followed by a fingle feed.

This is the form of the plant in whatever foil it grows. The diftinctions of the heath from the water Valerian are thefe.

The HEATH VALERIAN is about two feet and a half high. The ftalk is of a dufky green, and lightly hairy: the leaves are fmaller than in the water kind, and the little leaves of which each of the larger is compofed, are narrower, and of a deeper colour: thefe are alfo covered with fine white hairs. The flowers are of a brighter red; and the clufters of them are fmaller. The feed alfo is lefs.

The

The WATER VALERIAN is four feet high. The ftalk is of a pale green, and thick; the leaves are large, fmooth, and broad, and they are alfo of a frefh pale green. The flowers are paler; but larger, and more confpicuous than in the other; and the feed is larger and fofter.

This is the diftinction of the plants at full growth: but as the beft time of gathering the root is before the ftalk rifes, 'tis neceffary they fhould be known afunder alfo in that ftate. The place might indeed be a fufficient direction: for no one would go to gather the root by a river, when he has been told the Water Valerian is of lefs value. But that fuch as have not opportunities of taking it up themfelves, may have fome mark by which to know when it is genuine, it may be proper to add, that many fuch leaves as we have defcribed on the ftalk, rife alfo immediately from the root; and the fame diftinction is preferved in them: thefe in the Heath Valerian, are compofed of narrower parts, and are hairy and dufky in colour, in the Water Valerian, they are bright, fmoother, and pale.

The great diftinction is in the root itfelf. This in the true heath kind, is of a fine brown colour, tending to olive; and confifts of long flender fibres, which have a multitude of fmaller threads growing from their fides in the manner of fhort curled hairs. The root of the Wood Valerian is of a tawny or deep brownifh yellow.

The

The root of the Water Valerian, is of a pale brown tending to yellow ; and is compofed of thicker and more naked fibres : and there is lately introduced a kind which has grown in abfolute water. This is white, and is worft of all. The root of the Heath Valerian is firm and tough ; the root of the water kind is tender and more eafily broken : the Heath Valerian root has a frefh aromatick fcent, with a very little fœtidnefs. The water kind has nothing of this frefhnefs in the fcent, and little of the aromatick ; but is in a manner heavy and fœtid only.

By thefe characters the two plants will be known in whatever period of growth ; and even the roots when brought without any part of the plant. But as many have not opportunities of feeing thefe when frefh, it will be proper to obferve alfo its condition dry, at the druggifts. Thefe are fupplied with it by perfons who want knowledge, and often honefty : there is therefore no dependance, except upon the abfolute afpect of the drug. The diftinction in this article is the more neceffary ; becaufe the plant muft be wild to have its virtue. Garden culture debafes it almoft as much as a watery nourifhment abroad. This I have found by trial : and where a drug muft be received from fuch hands, as ufually deal in Valerian, it is neceffary to be very well acquainted with its genuine characters.

CHAP.

CHAP. III.

The History of the Valerian of the Druggists.

THE Valerian fold at our druggists is collected by a kind of itinerant medicine-mongers, whom from the principal article in which they deal, we call VIPER-CATCHERS: thefe people who travel over the greateft part of the kingdom in fearch of thofe animals, bring in alfo faffron, Valerian roots, and fome other articles.

As they find a hundred plants of the Water Valerian for one of the Heath or Wood kind, that is, the root they ufually collect: if the other falls in their way, and will come eafily out of the ground, as it will in the loofer heath foils after rains, they mix it with the reft: if not, they let it alone entirely: fo that we fometimes meet with great quantities of the water kind only; and fometimes with a mixture of one and the other. The firft fhould be refufed entirely, and the latter carefully picked. Befides this mixture, they put in alfo the roots of a fmall Meadow Valerian, a diftinct fpecies of plant: and others kind lefs pardonably. I have raifed a plant of the fmooth water crowfoot, which is poifonous, from a root fold among Wild Valerian.

Even this is not all the difadvantage. The time when root have then full virtue is before they fhoot up a ftalk; but this plant is moft obvious when in flower: the root alfo at that time

is

is loofer in the ground, and the ftalk is a handle by which it is eafily pulled up. For thefe rea-fons a great part of what is brought into the fhops has been taken out of the earth when the plant was in flower; and is therefore, even though the kind were right, unfit for ufe in medicine. Of all thefe imperfections the druggift fhould beware, for his care will make the gatherers honeft: if he be negligent, the apothecary fhould refufe to take fuch as is bad into his fhop; and in cafe of both thefe being carelefs, the patient may examine the root him-felf, according to the following characters.

C H A P. IV.

Defcription of the falfe Valerian Root when dry.

THE WATER VALERIAN ROOT dried is *brittle* and of a pale brown, approaching to *yellow* : it is compofed of many rounded fibres, often entirely *naked*, or at the beft hung with a very few threads; and at the head there are commonly feen the *remains* of a *ftalk*, with a hollow equal to that of a goofe quill. Among the true fibres of the root, are alfo feveral long and *thick ftrings* of a paler colour, and *jointed* as it were with a kind of dent at each joint. Thefe are the creeping appendages of the root, by which it runs under the furface: they have nearly the nature of ftalks, and are as defti-tute of virtue as fo many ftraws. When the real fibres are tafted, they are a little acrid, but *faint*, and a fœtid fcent is perceived in them while

C   chew-

chewing. If they are broken, they appear *hollow* in the midft, or at the beft dark and *blackifh*. In the firft cafe, the pith of the root is confumed, which is the common ftate of it it after the plant has flowered: the other is the natural condition of it in watery places, and the certain fign of its wanting ftrength. The fubftance which furrounds the pith in the Valerian root, contains its greateft virtue. This is fpungy and woody in the Water Valerian, but in the heath kind, it is firm, and contains a fubftance approaching to the nature of a gum-refin. This the watery nourifhment cannot fupply: and therefore this part in the Water Valerian is perifhable, which in the other is permanent.

C H A P. V.

Defcription of the true Heath Valerian Root when dry.

THE true Heath Valerian root is compofed of long and flender fibres: it is *tough* and of a *dufky brown*, approaching to *olive* colour; and the fibres are hung about with *numerous threads*. when broken, they have no hollow in the centre, nor any blackifh circle there, but appear full and bright; and if the root has been gathered in perfection, there is a circle of a greenifh or pale hue furrounding the pith.

The tafte differs from the other much more than the colour, or form: it is acrid, fpicy, and

pleafant

pleafant ; and after it has been chewed fome time, there is perceived a flight bitternefs and fome aftringency. It may be always known by this from the falfe ; which is vapid and fweetifh, fcarce at all aromatick, and deftitute entirely of this latent bitternefs and aftringency.

Its virtues depend wholly on the principles which give this tafte and favour, and they cannot be found in the other difagreeable and offenfive kind.

This is the root, and this only, which fhould be gathered for medicinal ufe, and it is indeed a very valuable and noble medicine. A phyfician of diftinguifhed abilities, one of the cenfors of the college *, has told me, that in a late fearch they found this true Valerian Root at one, and only one fhop in London ; the powder was of an olive brown, and the fcent aromatick and agreeable : at other places, the powder was of a yellowifh brown, and the fcent offenfive.

This true kind is liable like the falfe, to have runners mixed among the real fibres; and they fhould be feparated : it may be eafily feen whether the plant has been in ftalk at the time of its being gathered, and if it have, the root fhould be rejected 'Tis only in perfection when preparing to fhoot a ftem : and whoever will gather it at that time, will find this kingdom affords drugs equal to thofe of the warmeft climates.

* Dr Conier.

C 2   CHAP.

C H A P. VI.

Farther Trials of the two Roots.

VAlerian root is fometimes altered a little
in colour, from the foulnefs left about it
at the time of gathering; or from ill manage-
ment in drying. In this cafe, let fome of it
be put into cold water, and ftand twenty-four
hours. This never fails to diftinguifh the water from the heath kind; for the Water Valerian root becomes yellower, as it fwells, and
the other gets more of the olive brown than it
had while dry.

The fcent of the two roots alfo diftinguifhes
them; if they have not lain together : the true
is fragrant, though with a mixture of the fœtid
kind; the other abfolutely ftinks, and has fcarce
any thing of the aromatick fcent.

Cats, who have much more diftinguifhing
organs of fmell than we, perceive this. There
are certain fcents which affect them, and they
are principally of the fœtid kind; though this
is not without exception : they will bufy themfelves extremely about the Water Valerian root;
but fhew little regard to the other.

C H A P. VII.

Of gathering the Root.

THESE are the characters by which the
true Heath Valerian is to be known
from the falfe, ufually fold under its name.
When

When a parcel of this right kind is purchafed, before it is ufed, it fhould be picked ~~and~~ and cleaned: thofe roots which fhew they have borne a ftalk, are to be rejected; and the runners, or jointed and light ftrings muft be feparated from the true fibres. Thus the druggift will be fure he fells what the doctor prefcribes: but there ftill may remain a doubt about its value. The high flavour of the Valerian root is loft in long keeping, and the virtue in great part goes with it.

This root fhould never be ufed when it is more than one year old from the gathering: and the feller's word is not to be taken on this account, for he is always interefted to call the old new.

Under thefe difadvantages to which the purchafe of Valerian is fubjected on all hands, nothing can be fo rational as the patient's collecting it for himfelf. Where that cannot be done, let him be guided by the fame rules in the purchafe, that he would obferve in collecting it. Let him buy it frefh; at a right feafon of the year, and in the perfect ftate and condition: this he will know by the following rules.

Roots we fee poffefs their virtues in greateft perfection when they are ready for fhooting up a ftalk, but have not yet made the effort. 'Till that time they are imperfect, becaufe they have not obtained their full maturity, and after that they are exhaufted. The ultimate end of nature in the growth of plants, is the formation of the feeds: when thefe are perfected the

root

root is no longer ufeful: it becomes a ftick : and while the ftalk is in its growth, the rich juices are fent up fo faft to it, that the root is in great part drained of them. Therefore, neither when the plant is in flower, nor when it is about to flower, fhould its root be gathered for medicinal purpofes. While it has only the radical leaves it may: but the beft time of all is juft when the bud of the ftalk is forming.

The growth of the Valerian is this. In July it flowers ; in Auguft the feeds are ripe ; and the winds carrying them off, they ftrike root. The rains of autumn favour this; and a fmall clufter of leaves is formed: thefe, with the root, continue growing till the fevereft frofts ; or in mild winters through the whole feafon.

At the time when the feeds fall, thofe runners before-mentioned, rifing from the head of the old roots, fpread themfelves juft under the furface, or fometimes upon it, and taking root, they alfo form new plants. Each fhoots up a clufter of leaves, and fends fibres into the earth, juft as the feedlings

Among the roots we buy at the druggifts, fome are large and light ; others fmall and more firm : the large ones are often fuch as have been pulled up by the ftalk, at, or after the time of flowering, which are therefore in a great degree exhaufted. The fmall ones are the roots of feedling plants, and of thofe propagated by the runners. which have been taken up late in autumn, or early in fpring · and thefe having been in their earlieft ftate of growth, have not
their

their full virtue. This is the condition of the single roots brought to sale; and in the clusters of them, there is the greatest uncertainty: the larger part being exhausted, and often rotten; and the rest imperfect.

The true season for gathering Valerian root is the middle of May, and the finest are those of seedling plants. These are known by standing single; those from runners being always near old roots. These seedlings have had the autumn and winter for taking their first growth. The warmth and moisture of spring have now given them their full bigness, and toward the middle of May, the rudiment is formed, which is to shoot up into a stalk. The root is then full of its richest juice: and this is the proper season for gathering it.

In the system of vegetation, this is an universal truth: the root which has produced a stalk, and ripened flowers and seeds becomes an absolute chip, and has neither medicinal qualities, nor any other value. The purpose of nature is answered, and the whole plant dies. The MUSA will live a century if it does not flower, but when it has once bloom'd, no art can preserve it from immediate decay. The MOUNTAIN PALM, will live thirty or forty years barren; but if it flowers it instantly decays: and the TREE LAVATERA, which bears our winters even for many years till it blows, perishes as soon as that is over. Even annuals, by preventing their flowering, are kept alive thro' winter. In the bulbous kinds the root decays visibly, and in the others it has the same fate.

the root

though lefs obferved. The carrot which has run to feed, is an infipid ftick : and in the po- tatoe, though frefh roots are produced abun- dantly, that which was put into the ground in fpring, and which has borne the fummer ftalk is ufelefs.

The gardener thinks he takes up in July the fame bulb of the tulip, which he planted in November, but he deceives himfelf : that which he fets in autumn furnifhes the flower in the fucceeding fummer ; and, as it feeds the ftalk, decays. Another bulb is formed during this time, which contains the rudiment of the next year's flower : this encreafes as the other wi- thers ; and having attained its full growth by the middle of fummer, the gardener takes it up, and fuppofes it to be the fame he planted.

What we call a bulbous root is nothing more that a covering of the rudiment of the plant ; like the bud upon a tree : and the coats of the bulb, like the films, which compofe that bud, when they have perfoimed their office decay, and are renewed no more. The rudiment of the Valerian plant is a bud in the centre of the head of the root, of the fame kind with the other two ; and the root itfelf has the like fate. It naturally perifhes in the winter, when the plant has perfected its feeds ; and others are formed round about it, which fupply its place.

All this is tranfacted in the bofom of the earth, and at a time when roots are never taken up by the judicious : therefore it is little feen ; but it is the abfolute courfe of nature. The off-fets of bulbs, and the encreafed parts of

fibrous

Pl 2

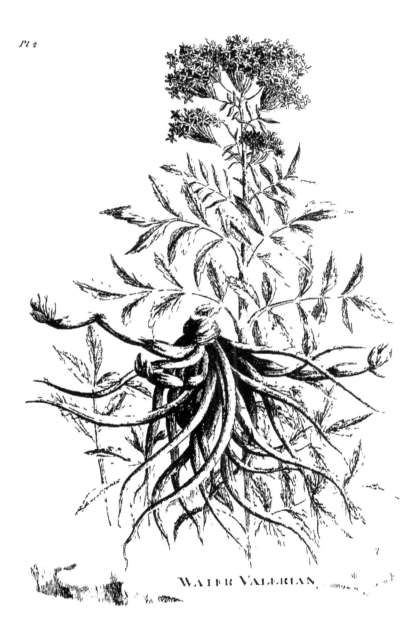

WATER VALERIAN.

fibrous roots, which the gardener feparates in parting them at autumn, are all formed in this manner ; containing the rudiments of new plants, and fupplying the place of the old roots, which decayed in flowering.

It is neceffary fo much fhould be known, to direct us in the proper gathering of roots ; and thus the philofophy of plants may ferve the pur-pofes of medicine.

C H A P. VIII.

The Manner of curing Valerian Root.

VALERIAN is in its greateft perfec-tion when frefh dried ; but the curing of medicinal roots, is a fubject we do not rightly manage in England. The *Ginfeng* of the Eaft-Indies, and the *Salep* of the Turks, are inftances that others have an art unknown to us. We cannot preferve any root as they do Ginfeng ; and with regard to Salep, our own Orchis would perfectly anfwer its purpofe, if we had the fame method of preparing it. This is not fo difficult as may be thought ; but it would be wandering from the prefent purpofe, to fpeak farther of the matter here.

When the Valerian roots are gathered, let the dirt be fhook from them, but not by ftriking them againft hard fubftances. It will feparate with little violence , and they muft neither be bruifed nor wafhed. Let the leaves and runners be cut off clean without wounding the head of the root, and then lay the whole

D   parcel

parcel in a heap in an airy place, where the
fun does not come: cover them with a blanket,
and leave them thus three days: then ftring
them up on long threads at ten inches diftance
root from root, and hang thefe threads acrofs
an airy room.

When they are perfectly dry, put them up
in boxes, prefling them clofe together, and covering them carefully.

Such as think laying the frefh root in heaps,
before it is hung up to dry, a ftrange practice,
may be reminded of the cuftom in regard to
fruits, whether intended for keeping, or for
wine. Thofe who underftand their manage-
ment, always give them a fweating of this
kind, for heightening their flavour, and im-
proving their natural qualities.

The gardener lays his pears in a heap, and
covers them with flannel, before he fpreads
them to keep for winter: and in the cyder countries, apples are treated in the fame manner before prefling; and in the wine countries, grapes.

A flight fermentation is thus brought on by
the warmth of the fubftances, and their flavour and virtues are exalted and improved. I
don't know that the fame practice has been ap-
plied to roots before, but the effect is fimilar;
and thofe who have not been accuftomed to Valerian otherwife than as feen in the fhops,
would fcaice fuppofe this the fame medicine:
it is highly aromatick, quick, and pungent on
the tongue, and the peculiar flavour in it, which
we call fœtid, fcaice deferves fo coarfe a name.

The

The root of Heath Valerian in this state poffeffes all the virtues which have been afcribed to
it by authors : it is a fovereign medicine in nervous diforders, and in particular exceeds all the
remedies commonly ufed againft that worft of
head-achs, which arifes from attention.

It has alone cured epilepfies : and of late it
has been ufed very fuccefsfully in hyfteric com-
plaints ; and in that terrible diforder the con-
vulfive afthma. It alleviates pain in the manner of the more gentle opiates ; and it is found
highly effectual in fits proceeding from the ob-
ftructions of the menfes; not only taking off the
fymptoms but removing the caufe. Perhaps
this root may be found, on experience, one of
the beft of our emmenagogues ; and I would
requeft thofe who have more opportunities to
try it farther in that intention.

A very large dofe of the frefh root will
purge ; but this is its leaft ufeful quality. I
have ordered it lately in that troublefome
difeafe the nightmare, and in two inftances,
wherein I have had fair opportunities to try
its virtue, have found it a perfect cure.

A very good method of taking it is frefh dried
in the way of tea, a dram of the root for a dofe,
with half a pint of boiling water; fweetened and
foftened with a little milk : but of all the pre-
parations, a tincture fully faturated with the in-
gredient muft be the beft. The root poffeffes its
full virtue only when it is frefh dried, after it has
been taken up at the feafon juft named. At that
time of the year it is excellent in powder, or in

the

the tea-infusion; but no method of keeping will preserve it in that perfect state : therefore the best recourse is to this form, and proof spirit is capable of receiving so strong a tincture from it, that a small dose will have great virtue. I have this year obtained from different parts of England a large quantity of the true root, and have found that an excellent tincture may be made from it in the following proportions.

Cut a pound and four ounces of the root just dried into small pieces, and bruise it in a mortar; put this into a gallon of proof-spirit, let it stand four days, shaking it every day, then strain off the liquor, pressing it hard. Put to this a pound of the root, bruised as before, and let it stand a week. after that strain and filter the tincture. A table spoonful is a dose.

I have made a quantity in this manner, which is at the service of my friends, or of the faculty; the rest of the root I have given to Mr. Tomson, a very worthy young man, who proposes to make it for the publick.

One farther improvement it is proper I name here, though sufficient experience has not yet confirmed me in its use: this is an ACID TINCTURE OF VALERIAN I have made this by adding two ounces of oil of vitriol to a pint of the preceding tincture, and have found it excellent: the acid exalts the flavour of the Valerian, and this tincture strengthens the stomach, creates an appetite, and always prevents that disorder of the head, to which nervous persons are subject after eating. The dose of the Valerian being

being limited by the acid, the plain tincture may be also taken at other times.

The roots fold by druggifts differ extremely in colour, tafte, fmell, and qualities; as they have been gathered in more or lefs favourable fituations and foils: the difference between the falfe and the true root, is that the one has grown in barren and dry ground; and the other in wet and muddy; and in confequence there are as many degrees of excellence or defect in the drug, as there are of foils between thofe two.

There are feveral parts of England, where the true kind is to be had in plenty. On the great heath called Hind-Head, in the road to Portfmouth, I have feen a vaft quantity of it; and Ray names it upon fufficient authority near Afhwood, by the Buxton-wells, in Derbyfhire; at Parnham, between Brindale and Orford, in Suffolk, and on Ilford Common.

The chief places whence the roots are brought for fale are four; the neighbourhood of Cambridge, the foreft of Dean in Gloucefterfhire, Oxford, and the near part of Kent. The Cambridge and Kentifh Valerian generally have a mixture of good and bad, for they pull up fome from the heaths and high grounds, which they mix among the water kind. what I have feen from about Oxford, has more of the Water Valerian; and from the foreft of Dean comes the pureft and beft our druggifts have · but this, like the reft, though the kind be better, is commonly taken up at a wrong feafon.

'Tis

'Tis faid none is imported : but I have found among parcels of it fome roots of a kind differ-ing in colour from almoft any of the Eng-lifh forts; and alfo the tuberous white roots of the nardus montana radice olivari, which is a vale-rian, not native of this kingdom ; therefore thofe parcels of the drug probably came from France, and could not but be worfe for the keeping : it does not appear that any part of the world pro-duces this drug in greater perfection than our own country, provided the foil and fituation be proper.

That foil, and fituation, can make fo con-fiderable a difference in the virtues of plants, appears from various inftances in nature; and as plainly from the effects of culture. Lavender and other aromatick herbs, are fweeter, and fuller of virtue in thofe kingdoms where they grow wild, than with us who raife them only in gardens ; and many which we have wild in common with the fouth of France, are yet greatly fuperior in their qualities there.

Culture renders the common garden plants larger and more fucculent; but it takes off their tafte and qualities : and the difference between the Heath and Water Valerian is very like that of a wild and garden herb ; the fituation in the muddy bank of a ditch, giving abundant moi-fture and nourifhment.

We fee the fame plant is more richly fla-voured when it grows in a dry foil, and more infipid when in wet. and we find the higheft aromaticks are natives of dry and
with

warm lands: indeed to know the effect of abundant moifture and rich earth, we need look no farther than the common lettuce. In the wild ftate, wherein it lives on dry, parched, and barren ground, its juice is acrid and bitter, and its virtue highly narcotick; fo much as to have obtained it the name of poifonous: in gardens where it has rich mould, and abundant moifture, it becomes mild, pleafant, and innocent. Nor does the form differ lefs: when wild the ftalk is woody, and the leaves are prickly: when cultivated the ftem is tender, and the leaves are unarmed. So the auftere crab of the common, becomes the mellow apple of the orchard; and the bitter almond, fweet.

The cafe is the fame in all thefe inftances: the virtues or the qualities of the herb, root, or fruit, depend upon the natural and moderate quantity of juices elaborated, undifturbed in the veffels; and well concocted by the fun: this gives the tafte, fcent, flavour, and medicinal qualities. When nature throws its feeds in a rich wet foil, or human induftry removes them to the garden, the character of the plant is altered, the effective particles are debafed or drowned among the additional quantity of juice, and the whole becomes in the end taftelefs, fcentlefs, inefficacious, and infipid.

On thefe principles the culture of the Valerian muft never be attempted; and in its wild ftate, fo much depends upon the nature of the foil and feafon of the year, that it is happy the characters of excellence and imperfection

fection are marked so strongly on the root itself.
Those who neglect to observe them will be disappointed in their expectations from this drug,
though in reality it possesses all the virtue that
has been ascribed to it; and deserves more com-
mendation than has been given even by its
warmest advocates.

THE END.

Directions for placing the PLATES,

CPSIA information can be obtained
at www.ICGtesting.com
Printed in the USA
BVHW061353270619
552120BV00012B/318/P